WAKE UP, AMERICA

By

Gene Cordes

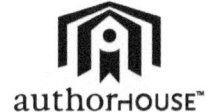
authorHOUSE™

1663 LIBERTY DRIVE, SUITE 200
BLOOMINGTON, INDIANA 47403
(800) 839-8640
WWW.AUTHORHOUSE.COM

First published by AuthorHouse 3/30/2005
Revised 11/12/2007

ISBN: 1-4208-0335-2 (sc)

Library of Congress Control Number: 2007909472

Printed in the United States of America
Bloomington, Indiana

This book is printed on acid-free paper.

This revision is dedicated to my wife of sixty years, a former Lady Marine, who almost singlehandedly raised our three children due to my extensive travels as a Federal Auditor.

INTRODUCTION

We are the greatest superpower on the face of the earth, but our democracy has a lot to be desired due to Corporate America controlling our lives via campaign contributions. Medical experts have cited building materials that offgas hazardous chemicals causing cancer and other illnesses, but lack effective controls to please Corporate America. We cannot afford National Health Insurance coverage until we have chemical controls in place for an extended period.

We must return to government of the people, by the people and for the people. No greater need for this exists except in housing where Corporate America, via contributions, dictate our housing regulations in spite of consumer complaints.

This is corruption, pure and simple. To digress for a moment, greed and corruption destroyed the Roman and Greek empires, and is suspected of destroying the empire of the Soviet Union after seventy years of communism.

Only a flood of mail to Senators and Congressmen by the readers can change all this with a citation of "Wake Up, America"!

With the Supreme Court's decision on December 10, 2003, there is great hope for the future – by a narrow margin of 5 to 4, the Court upheld the new campaign-finance law which banned "soft-money" donations to national political parties and prohibited interest groups from running issue ads immediately before Federal elections. The law that President Bush signed in March of 2002 will supposedly govern all future presidential and congressional elections."

****** The author wished to acknowledge the source of the quotations on pages 5 & 6 from the book entitled "An Alternative Approach to Allergies" by Theron G. Randolph, M.D. and Ralph W. Moss, Ph.D. Copyright 1980. Reprinted by permission of HarperCollins Publishers, Inc., 10 East 53rd Street, New York, N.Y. 10022.

TABLE OF CONTENTS

PART I – HUD & EPA: PUPPETS OF THE INDUSTRIAL LOBBY

Preface

Since we are all structured differently, we react differently when exposed to chemicals in the home or workplace. One example of this occurred during the Vietnam War, i.e., not all soldiers suffered permanent injury when exposed to the defoliant Agent Orange, but many did have permanent injuries, mental and/or physical, due to longtime exposure. The sad part of the story is that, for many years, the government refused to treat these illnesses as war-related, and when it was finally determined to be related, many veterans were deceased. This allowed for a relatively smaller

*

---

* HUD is the U.S. Dept. of Housing Urban Development; EPA is the U.S. Environmental Protection Agency.

1

budget amount to be applied to these illnesses – a fact that makes one wonder if this was what the government sought from the start. Moreover, there was a chemical exposure during the Gulf War that left many service people no longer able to serve, but again, the government stalled in providing treatment for these service-connected disabilities. Finally, when treatment was provided, it appeared to be with the knowledge that the budget amount would not be overwhelming.

Damning Evidence Against HUD and EPA

The background to the 1984 HUD regulation for Manufactured Home Construction and Safety Standards, contained in Volume 49, Federal Register 31996-32003 dated 8/9/84, shows damning evidence that HUD and EPA were controlled by the industrial lobby, and the consumer comments were ignored. Section I-D of that background describes a National Manufactured Home Advisory Council of 24 members divided equally among industry, government agencies, and consumer groups. That section also describes three days of workshop sessions by council subcommittees held in September 1983 with related reports available for public inspection. However, when I requested a review of the reports in October 1993, I was informed that they were destroyed. This was highly unusual destruction since ten years had not elapsed since the 8/9/84 issuance date of the regulation.

Section II-B-1 of the background states that State agencies endorsed the use of an ambient standard that would limit the level of formaldehyde in the home and ensure maintenance of a safe level of that chemical in the home by limiting outgassing from all sources of the chemical used in the home's construction. However, Section II-B-2 states that the manufactured home industry (industrial lobby) especially endorsed the use of a product standard which is precisely what HUD required, i.e., a pre-construction product standard requiring that formaldehyde emissions not exceed 0.2 parts per million (ppm) from plywood and 0.3 ppm from particleboard. Thus, the manufactured home industry was protected from claims regarding homes that have high levels of formaldehyde. Section II-C-1 states that "A number of consumers and academic sources stated that it was imperative that the plywood standard be lowered." Section II-C-2 states that "The response from consumers and several other sources on the particleboard standard was much like the response to the plywood standard." Also, that section states that "A few consumers felt that urea-formaldehyde-based particleboard was so significant an emitter that it should be banned from use in manufactured homes." However, HUD ignored these consumers and academic sources. Section II-D states that "The Department (HUD) has concluded that an indoor ambient formaldehyde level of 0.4 ppm provides reasonable protection to manufactured home occupants." Section II-D-2 also states that "The Department will reevaluate the formaldehyde standards when the EPA reaches a final regulatory decision and may change the standards if the basis for EPA's finding show that these standards are not adequate to protect the health of manufactured home occupants." (See Exhibit A) In 1987, EPA concluded that formaldehyde is "a probable human carcinogen", but has taken no meaningful action since to control the hazardous substance.

Dr. Thad Godish of Ball State University issued a paper in 1989 citing formaldehyde as a potent eye, upper respiratory and skin irritant; and a cause of headaches, fatigue and depression. He also lists 28 possible symptoms/health problems that could result from such exposure, including disturbed concentration. In addition, he cites the residential indoor air quality standard of 0.1 ppm maximum concentration for the chemical in Germany and the Netherlands, and a recommended action level of 0.1 ppm for residential exposure in Canada; and NASA's standard of 0.1 ppm for manned space travel since 1967. In comparison, he cites the lack of an indoor air quality standard for the chemical in the U.S., and adds that release of the chemical from source materials "will never completely stop."

To placate consumer groups, HUD's 1984 regulation required a health warning on display for new home sales citing children, elderly and allergy/asthma sufferers as being at greater risk. However, HUD has not provided for spot checks at dealer locations for this health warning, as contained in Title 24 of the Code of Federal Regulations, Section 3280.309, as of 8/9/84. Moreover, on 5/17/99, HUD Asst. Secretary Hal C. DeCell III advised me in response to a Congressional Inquiry, that "... the Department has consistently recommended to all participating State agencies that they implement a dealer monitoring program, (but) only a certain number of States have chosen to do so... As such, there is little we can do, except to strongly recommend to the State, as we have done, that it provide a more exhaustive consumer protection program." Thus, HUD is not enforcing its own regulation, even on a spot check basis, throughout the 50 states. (See Exhibit B)

Medical Experts

Dr. Theron Randolph founded the American Academy of Environmental Medicine. His book entitled "An Alternative Approach to Allergies" details his sweeping challenge to orthodox medical thinking, and was first issued in 1980, but later revised in 1989. He stated in his revised edition that "From my viewpoint, however, the cancer-causing potential of formaldehyde, although highly important, is only part of the story. The second, and possibly more important, formaldehyde story is the immediate and long-term effects of this chemical on the mental and physical health of millions of people." He drives his point home when he states "It is difficult to ignore your neighbor, for instance, who is sleeping in a tent in the backyard because she cannot live with the fumes of formaldehyde outgassing from the particle board in her house!" He also related the problem to conventional as well as manufactured homes. In that connection, the definition of a "Manufactured Home" contained in the HUD regulation exempts all modular homes that use the same materials as manufactured homes, by insertion of the phrase "on a permanent chassis". Thus, thousands, and possibly millions, of modular homes are exempt from the regulation even though they contain similar materials as found in manufactured homes on a permanent chassis. Likewise, conventional homes contain the same basic health-threatening materials.

A study by Drs. Ritchie and Lehnen, reported in the 1987 American Journal of Public Health, covered 2,000 residents in mobile and conventional homes in the state of Minnesota; and concluded that the HUD "target level" of 0.4 ppm may not be adequate to protect occupants from acute effects of formaldehyde exposure. The HUD "target level" was explained in the background to the 1984 regulation as providing reasonable protection from all formaldehyde sources including plywood and particleboard that are subject to preconstruction product standards.

However, this "target level" is still four times that recommended by medical experts and set forth as a standard or recommended level in three foreign countries.

In 1984, the California Dept. of Health Services stated "Viewed strictly from the standpoint of health risk from formaldehyde exposure, no evidence has been educed that would justify advocating a level higher than 0.05 parts per million (ppm) detection limit for field measurements." (220 California Reporter 712-720, 1985)

The Minnesota Dept. of Health stated in March 1991 that "the most common guideline for acceptable formaldehyde levels is 0.1 ppm."

Other Experts

The American Society of Heating, Refrigerating, and Air-Conditioning Engineers, and the American Industrial Hygiene Association recommended a maximum concentration of 0.1 ppm (per Environmental Science and Technology, August 1989).

In the fall of 1999, I called most of the major carpet manufacturers in Dalton, Ga., where an estimated 60 percent of all carpet produced in the world is made within a 50-mile radius of this city. I inquired as to their use of formaldehyde in the manufacturing process, and was informed that they have now substituted "4 Phenylcyclohexene", a/k/a "4-PC". This chemical was cited in "The Human Ecologist" published in the Spring of 1993 by the Human Ecology Action League (HEAL) of Atlanta, GA., as having been tested by the Anderson Laboratories, Inc., of Dedham, MA., with fumes from small carpet samples resulting in eight mouse fatalities of the nine tests conducted. CBS Evening News also gave prime-time coverage of the carpet controversy, quoting a consumer whose children became ill after a home carpet installation, as also reported by HEAL in 1993. In contrast, Shaw Industries, Inc., of Dalton, Ga., a leading carpet manufacturer using "4-PC", states in a 7-page dissertation that "Odor is well recognized as a very important factor in the perception of Indoor Air Quality. Odors perceived as bad or harmful can induce stress and anxiety. Symptoms such as headache and nausea can result." In other words, the consumer is imagining a problem! Needless to say, EPA has taken no meaningful action to control the chemical.

A Common Thread Causing Illness?

A chemist advised me that formaldehyde is also a component of wood combustion, tobacco smoke, or a part of the metabolic process. Thus, it is important to ventilate indoor areas and avoid the cumulative effect of building materials, wood smoke and/or tobacco smoke.

As an example, the Meredith Publishing Co. released a Family Medical Guide in 1966 that stated "...certain drugs and chemicals, if administered to normal people, will within two weeks produce in them all the symptoms of Parkinson's Disease. The fact that chemical substances can produce Parkinson symptoms in normal people indicates that the immediate cause of true Parkinson's disease must be toxic chemical substances, as yet unidentified...and gradually produce tremor, rigidity, and slowness of movement." The toxic substances could conceivably be formaldehyde and/or "4-PC" that reduce the body's resistance to a variety of other conditions that the medical community finds difficult or impossible to treat!

State of Wisconsin defeated by the HUD Regulation

The State of Wisconsin attempted to legislate more stringent control over formaldehyde in manufactured homes only to be defeated in the case of Liberty Homes, Inc. vs. Dept. of Industry, Labor and Human Relations, 374 N.W. 2nd 142 (Wis. 1985) affirmed, 401 N.W. 2nd 805 (1987), since the court specifically held that the applicable Federal Regulation preempted a State rule establishing a maximum permissible formaldehyde concentration in the indoor air of new manufactured homes offered for sale in Wisconsin. Thus, the industrial lobby's control over HUD and EPA is far-reaching, but must be reversed to overcome illnesses to millions of consumers!

Potential Effect

The potential effect from formaldehyde offgassing alone can be measured by HUD's own health warning for manufactured homes that was inserted in the 1984 regulation to placate consumer groups. The warning states "Elderly persons and young children, as well as anyone with a history of asthma, allergies, or lung problems, may be at greater risk." The 2000 census shows 19.2 million children under 5 years old, and 35 million persons 65 years old and older. Both these categories total 54.2 million person, or approximately 19.3% of the total population of 280.4 million.

Also, while overlapping these categories to some extent, U.S. Healthcare estimated in 1991 that 20 percent of the population has allergies – this extrapolates to 56.1 million persons when applied to the 2000 census. (See Exhibit B for health warning)

Thus, millions are at risk with formaldehyde exposure in the home, especially when the offgassing allowed is four times as much as recommended by medical experts, and set forth as a standard or recommended level in three foreign countries, i.e., 0.1 ppm recommended by medical experts of held as a standard or recommended level in three foreign countries, versus 0.4 ppm "target level" mentioned by HUD in the background to the 1984 regulation with EPA concurrence, and still standing in spite of the 1987 conclusion by EPA that the chemical is "a probable human carcinogen".

Personal Experience

After purchasing a manufactured home in Florida in 1988 that lacked the Federally-required health warning on display, I suffered with headaches, fatigue, depression, and bronchitis. I fitted two of the health warning categories, i.e., elderly and allergy sufferers. After vacating the home, I have continued to suffer with permanent liver damage, more severe sensitivity to most medications, both prescription and off-the-shelf. The latter is now life-threatening with high blood pressure medications having severe side effects.

When I discovered the health warning several months after moving into the manufactured home and requiring heat one night, I placed a notice in the village newsletter advising occupants to ventilate their manufactured home if away during the summer. One resident called to inform me that he now understood why he had to visit his cardiologist for medication after spending the summer in upstate New York. He had never ventilated upon returning and faced the cumulative effect of the toxic offgassing!

After vacating the manufactured home in 1991, I was unable to take vitamin pills for six years because of headaches. In 1997, when I was diagnosed with prostate cancer, I returned to vitamin pills without having headaches. The vitamin D contained therein prevented the spread of the cancer until 2002 when the "PSA" reading jumped from below "7.8" to "10.5". I learned after receiving radiation that a sudden upward reading could be caused by an infection.

However, without knowing this, I agreed to hormonal treatment and radiation without the urologist, Dr. Michael Naslund of the U. of Md. Medical Center in Baltimore even double-checking the "PSA" test before proceeding. Before proceeding, another biopsy revealed the same prostate condition as in 1997, i.e., one of six specimens contained cancer.

I received 84 radiation seeds on December 9, 2002. The urologist visited my hospital room the following morning and advised that "stones" were removed from my bladder during the operation. I had no history of bladder problems, but an oncologist-friend advised that some of the seeds may have missed the prostate target and lodged in the bladder, requiring removal and replacement in the prostate. At approximately 2 P.M. on December 10, 2002, I was visited by a Doctor Gupta in my hospital room who handed me two prescriptions for pain and an anti-biotic, and a followup appointment slip, and then advised me "You are discharged".

My son picked me up at the curb outside the hospital shortly thereafter.

Pain intensified after taking two pain pills six hours later, so I called several hospital numbers until I reached a Doctor on duty and explained my history and condition. He advised me to take a third or fourth pain pill and that ended the telecom. We both apparently thought the pain was caused by radiation. A third pain pill gave me no relief so I dialed "911" and an ambulance picked me up ten minutes later and delivered me to the Anne Arundel Medical Center in Annapolis 30 minutes later. I felt I was near death in the ambulance and was given an injection at a stop along the way. The hospital immediately inserted a catheter that relieved me of 1300 cc. of urine that had caused the pain. My blood pressure had reached 251/106 due to the pain, and if it were not for my cardiac arrhythmia since birth that prevented excessive weight, I would have had a stroke or died. Nevertheless, I had a complete occlusion of my left eye (peripheral vision only) and a mildly dilated aortic root that requires monitoring. During the ambulance trip, it occurred to me that I had not urinated for some time and that my urinary tract must be blocked by swelling of my prostate, and that had to cause the hyperventilation due to the pain, and thus, damaging effects.

I was unable to obtain medical support for a malpractice lawsuit, so I resorted to filing a seven-page complaint with the Maryland Board of Physicians and attached twelve exhibits. My complaint was filed in March of 2005. Two pages of rebuttal by the urologist that contained many false statements resulted in the Board's closing of the file in September of 2005. The urologist's statement did not require any certification as to the truth. The truth is this: I would not have risked my life if I had been warned at any time that the prostate could enlarge and block the urinary tract, thus requiring re-catheterization. Moreover, a series of reports in the Baltimore Sun from December 12 through December 22, 2005, concluded that the Board only reviews those doctors with three malpractice settlements of $150,000 each over five years or those who settle a case for $1 million or more.

A further conclusion should be that Public Law 99-660 entitled "Health Care Quality Improvement Act of 1986" is a failure in many, if not all, states since it apparently has not been effective in removing incompetent physicians. My personal experience can be summed up as follows:

1. My wife and I inspected five villages in Florida with an average of ten models in each one, and never saw the Federally-required health warning in

any of them. We unknowingly chose a Palm Harbor manufacturer because of the excellent design, but all of their homes contained Particleboard resulting in a severe case of bronchitis when the heat was turned on.

2. The exposure to formaldehyde prevented me from taking vitamin D for nine years without headaches. Once a biopsy showed cancer, I again tried the vitamin in 1997 without having a headache. The sudden increase in the PSA reading in 2002 led me to radiation treatment, but a later news release explained any sudden increase to a possible infection. There was no attempt by the Baltimore hospital to double-check the sudden increase, but an infection could have held it high.

3. The poor choice of a Baltimore hospital for treatment of one cancerous prostate specimen out of six, and agreeing to hormonal and radiation treatment that I felt was necessary at the time, but probable not requiring 84 radiation seeds, resulted in a near-death situation for lack of proper warning by the urologist before discharge from the hospital, and the doctor on duty six hours later who merely instructed me to take a third or fourth pain pill when I really needed re-catheterization. The latter felt as I did apparently that it was radiation-related pain.

4. Finally, the lack of enforcement of the required health warning at dealer locations by Federal authorities was the beginning of my many health problems that continue today.

PART II – PRESIDENT CLINTON'S 1998 EXECUTIVE ORDER JEOPARDIZED THE LIVES OF FEDERAL WORKERS

Preface

To understand how President Clinton could sign an Executive Order jeopardizing the lives of Federal workers, one must summarily review his administration's eight years of "anything goes", as follows:

1. Richard Miniter authored a book entitled "Losing bin Laden: How Bill Clinton's Failures Unleashed Global Terror" in which he describes the number of missed opportunities he had to capture and imprison or kill the terrorist leader Osama bin Laden,

but instead, we are sill hunting him after the four-plane hijacking/destruction on 9/11/01 and ten-plane attempted but foiled hijacking in Great Britain reported on 8/11/06. In one instance in 1996, Sudan's Minister of State offered to arrest and turn over bin Laden and asked "Where should we send him?", but a CIA official stated "We have nothing we can hold him on." The author points out that the Clinton foreign policy was to get re-elected, and therefore, anything that might be controversial had to be avoided.

2. In 2004, Attorney General John Ashcroft testified before the September 11 Commission that the Clinton administration's FBI technology budget through September 30, 2001 was actually $36 million less than the last Bush budget eight years before, thus hampering tracking of terrorists, and also taking aim at one of the September 11 Commissioners for creating a "wall" in 1995 between law enforcement and intelligence gathering.

3. On his last day in office in 2001, President Clinton pardoned Marc Rich for a scheme described by authorities as one of the biggest tax fraud cases in U.S. history involving the funnelling of over $70 million to Swiss banks from illegal profits due to the resale of crude oil.

4. Columnist Oliver North described Clinton's defense of pre-9/11 actions during a Fox interview in September 2006 as violations of three Executive Orders in 1976, 1978 and 1981 barring political assassinations. Clinton stated in that interview "I worked hard to try to kill him (Osama bin Laden). I authorized a finding for the CIA to kill him. We contracted with people to kill him. I got closer to killing him than anybody has gotten since."

5. Last but not least, President Clinton had a scandalous relationship with a young White House intern, Monica Lewinsky, whom he charged with lying, but her soiled dress proved otherwise.

Clinton's Executive Order in 1998

The Preface was intended to summarize the Clinton administration's "anything goes" policy that applied with the signing of Executive Order 13101 entitled "Greening the Government through Waste Prevention, Recycling, and Federal Acquisition". The General Services Administration (GSA) implemented the policy contained in the Executive Order, and the Environmental Protection Agency (EPA), guardian of our environment, issued comprehensive guidelines for furniture procurements, including furniture made with particleboard. As mentioned previously under the caption "Damning Evidence Against HUD and EPA", EPA concluded in 1987 that formaldehyde is "a probable human carcinogen", but nevertheless permitted recycling of particleboard manufactured in a bath of formaldehyde and recycled with a fresh bath to produce desks, chairs, file cabinets and closets. Such furniture might just as well be tagged "Welcome Federal employees to a slow death". To make the connection, the reader need only refer to the Exhibit entitled "Occupant Symptom/Health Problem Checklist" authored by Prof. That Godish of Ball State University and re-printed with his permission. The 28-point checklist, once followed according to the instructions, could be a clear indication of chemical sensitivity caused by the recycled particleboard furniture, and the need for Federal managers to take corrective action, not only to revise the Executive Order and implementing orders, but to replace existing furniture with safe open market furniture.

One particular case of recycled particleboard for office furniture caught my attention. A large group of Department of Defense employees looked forward to moving into a new building and vacating a very old building in Arlington, Virginia, in the spring of 2005. Alas, the new building was filled with various office furniture made with recycled particleboard. Very few of the employees could afford expensive air filters that extract formaldehyde offgassing from the particleboard furniture. In addition, only small offices could deal with the purification process, since open bays are impossible to control via individual air filters. Moreover, building ventilating systems are shut down after work hours and on weekends. Therefore, employees working overtime in the evenings or weekends are subject to higher density offgassing of formaldehyde. Moreover, the objective of saving electricity after regular work hours and weekends is overcome by the many debilitating effects of breathing higher density fumes, notably, less productivity due to various ill feelings. In that connection, seven of the 28 possible effects from the chemical exposure are described on page 4 as set forth by Dr. Thad Godish of Ball State University in his pamphlet issued in 1989. The importance of this subject is emphasized by the quote from Dr. Theron Randolph's book contained on page 5, i.e, the cancer-causing potential and the immediate and long-term effects of formaldehyde on the mental and physical health of millions of people. For a more detailed explanation of the shortcomings of EPA in controlling formaldehyde, the reader should refer to the eight pages contained in the 1989 revision of Dr. Randolph's book entitled "An Alternative Approach to Allergies" that leaves no doubt that corporations control EPA instead of EPA protecting the consumer. One expert quoted by Dr. Randolph described the exposure as "classical chemical susceptibility" and the writer recommends tracking of the revised edition through Harper Collins Publishers of New York.

PART III - OBSERVATIONS

A. Made in China

A cable telecast in November, 2006, reported that China manufactures particleboard for export to the United States, but forbids its use in constructing homes for its 1.2 billion population in communist China. If this is true, then China protects its citizens from health problems, while the government of the United States protects Corporate America from lawsuits, i.e., by permitting excessive chemical offgassing resulting in unhealthy homes that lack a proper indoor air standard, and that same government, Executive and Legislative branches, is rewarded with campaign contributions to all major political parties and candidates fro public office. (Ref: "Damning Evidence against HUD & EPA" found in Part I).

In that regard, National Committees are permitted $26,700 annually for each Committee and from each donor; and individual candidates are permitted $2,100 annually for each candidate and from each donor. These limits allow sufficient leverage for Corporate America to control Federal Regulations as at present lacking proper indoor air standards. Thousands, and possibly millions of people have been subject to cancer and other illnesses resulting in death over the years, and because of the 1984 HUD regulation described in Part I for manufactured homes, and the lack of protection for conventionally-built homes having the same health problems described in Part I. Wake up, America!

B. Asthma epidemic in children

A 1999 news item reported that EPA would host a two-day conference at Johns Hopkins University on how to fight childhood asthma, a respiratory disease that has reached epidemic proportions and afflicts almost 5 million children nationwide. The host is partly to blame for the epidemic! While not directly related, a news item in the past year reported that the cancer rate was declining. By a stretch of the imagination, could this be because of the trend by builders and renovators to use laminated flooring in place of carpeting that in the past has contained harmful chemicals used for adhesives?

Finally, EPA Administrator Stephen Johnson is currently the first scientist to lead EPA, and as such, will he be the first to rein in harmful chemical offgassing with an indoor air standard? To close this observation with a chuckle, the National Particleboard Association (NPA) funded a research effort by EPA concerning particleboard, but when headed for an unwelcome conclusion for NPA, NPA refused to provide additional funds. Foot dragging continued by EPA through 1997 with no current reading on its status.

C. Dealer locations and health warnings

In response to a Congressional Inquiry on my behalf in 2005, HUD Assistant Secretary Steven Nesmith states that HUD has "always monitored factories and retailer lots for compliance with the Construction and Safety Standards, including the Health Notice requirement. In fact, since the beginning of 2005, this process has identified five manufactured homes in which the Health Notice was not properly posted or was missing."

However, this statement does not mention the universe in which the Health Notice was found missing. Also, since the term "always" suggests "forever and a day", why did I miss seeing one health warning in 1989 after visiting five Florida villages containing about fifty model homes, and as a result, purchased one home containing formaldehyde in particleboard and carpeting? As a matter of fact, during the three year period of ownership, the Armstrong Corporation replaced all of the floor tile in the kitchen, bath and laundry room of the "Palm Harbor" type purchased because the particleboard adhesive had seeped into the tile from the particleboard subfloor. I am not aware of how many "Palm Harbor" types existed in the 750 home village, but it was an extensive project cost apparently to be borne by the particleboard or home manufacturer. Since I had not registered the complaint, I am not aware of the outcome. This story emphasizes the need to enforce the Health Notice requirement. The lack of the Health Notice in my situation resulted in extensive health problems that continue today. Notwithstanding, if an indoor air standard existed and was enforced, there would be no need for the warning.

D. Witness to the persecution of individuals

A close co-worker and veteran of World War II retired from the Federal Government in 1979, and moved to a suburb of Savannah, Georgia. He lived in a beautiful new rambler there and eventually suffered a mild stroke while his wife underwent a double mastectomy. His active lifestyle including golf was restricted so they bought a new townhouse nearby. Once again, he suffered a mild stroke. They placed their names on a waiting list with 300 other names ahead of them at the Forest at Duke retirement home near Duke University Medical Center at Durham, North Carolina. Eventually, their names were called up, their townhouse was sold, and they moved into their apartment at the retirement home.

We visited them in their apartment several years ago and they discussed their plans to renovate it with new carpet. They implemented their plan and renovated with new carpet. In December of 2005, we received a letter from his wife advising that she lost her husband in the previous month, and that the doctors at Duke Medical Center cared for him for a week before he died, but "couldn't find out just what was wrong". This reminds me of my first exposure to formaldehyde in our manufactured home in Florida. I visited five doctors before the fifth one, an allergy specialist, was familiar with chemical offgassing, and offered suggestions to relieve the symptoms, In the case of my co-worker and his wife suffering health problems in new living quarters, you can bet your bottom dollar that the fresh carpet was the cause, and it had to contain formaldehyde or "4-PC" as described in Part I.

Another situation involved a visit to my cousin in Laguna Beach, California, in 1999. He had suffered a stroke seven months before and had to be placed in a nursing home. He asked me to take him for a visit to his home at the top of the mountain where he lived alone. When we arrived there, I gasped for breath as soon as I entered, and immediately opened windows to remove the cumulative offgassing from new carpet. I asked when he had it installed, and he said "Last February". Then I asked when he had his stroke and he replied "In March". Case closed. Another victim of HUD and EPA serving corporate America instead of protecting the public. A third situation involved my son purchasing a townhouse in 1995 with fresh "Shaw" carpeting. Each time I would visit, I would ventilate the house to avoid the cumulative offgassing from the carpet. After six years, the "half-life" or most dangerous offgassing was over, as described by Professor Godish in his 1989 paper, and described further in Part I. Moreover, a 2006 telephone survey revealed that "Shaw", "Mohawk", and "Alladin" carpet manufacturers had switched to "synthetic latex" as an adhesive, and joined "Berber" in producing safe carpeting.

It is conceivable that the foregoing changes resulted from delivery of my 2005 book edition to the HUD Secretary and the EPA Administrator in the Spring of 2005.

If the reader should suspect an unhealthy home situation, Dr. That Godish's "Occupant Symptom/ Health Problem Checklist" shown at Exhibit C should be utilized to make a determination as to whether or not a problem exists.

A recent event just came to my attention involving a friend who purchased a $700,000 modular home in the Boston area about two years ago. She has suffered two heart attacks that apparently stemmed from the particleboard construction. As mentioned previously, modular homes do not come within the purview of the HUD regulation since the definition of a manufactured home includes the phrase "on a permanent chassis" and even though such homes contain the same cheap materials as found in the so-called "mobile" or "manufactured" home. Credit Corporate America with the addition of this phrase by HUD in framing the 1984 regulation.

E. Warnings to Congressmen that were ignored

In September of 2005, the news media reported that 300,000 trailer homes were being ordered for Katrina hurricane survivors. Knowing very well that manufacturers would maximize their profits by using particleboard instead of plywood, and that the carpeting would probably contain "4-PC" as described in Part I, I wrote warning letters to Rep. William J. Jefferson of Louisiana, and Rep. Robert Aderholt of Alabama calling their attention to the plight of hurricane survivors who would be faced with offgassing and health problems in the new trailers. Both congressmen ignored my warnings even though Rep. Aderholt serves on both the HUD and the EPA appropriation subcommittees. As a consequence, the residents suffering illnesses are seeking individual lawsuits against the Federal Government and the trailer manufacturers. This lawsuit is aided by subpoenaed records by a Congressional committee in July 2007 that showed the Federal Emergency Management Agency (FEMA) lawyers advised against further testing of trailers for fear of potential liability problems, notwithstanding the deaths of two trailer occupants and numerous illnesses/complaints.

PART IV - PREFACE TO RECOMMENDATIONS

There are many building materials containing formaldehyde used in the construction of manufactured and conventional homes, but the foremost ones are plywood and particleboard. This is why HUD required a pre-construction product standard for these two materials; i.e., formaldehyde emissions not to exceed 0.2 ppm from plywood and 0.3 ppm from particleboard. However, these standards are too high for a healthy home, and the so-called "target level" for indoor air of 0.4 ppm is too high, but because it is a "target level", it prevents builders from being sued even if this level is exceeded. As mentioned earlier, there must be an indoor air standard of 0.1 ppm maximum concentration for formaldehyde exposure as found in certain foreign countries and as found in NASA's standard for manned space travel since 1967. Such a standard can be attained by a vacuum process.

Similarly, such a standard must be set for the carpet industry that had apparently substituted "4-PC" for formaldehyde that is just as detrimental to health as formaldehyde as previously stated. Testing for "4-PC" should be possible in a manner similar to formaldehyde, and a vacuum process should make it attainable.

As mentioned in Part I – "Damning Evidence Against HUD and EPA", Dr. Godish states that release of formaldehyde from source materials "will never completely stop", but a half-life of about 5 or 6 years, depending on temperature and humidity, should be the maximum health threat under the existing "target level". An indoor air standard of 0.1 ppm maximum concentration of these hazardous chemicals should significantly aid in providing healthy indoor air for family members, and this is our goal for both manufactured and conventional homes – even though Congress has only had an interest in manufactured homes in the past. The study by Drs. Ritchie and Lehnen described in Part I demonstrated that residents of both manufactured and conventional homes suffer health problems from formaldehyde exposure and both areas much have the aforementioned indoor air standard to protect our family members from cancer and other illnesses.

Please note that the present HUD definition of manufactured homes must be revised to include "modular" homes. Also note the contents of Exhibit A whereby consumers were ignored by HUD in formulating the 1984 regulation. Moreover, Exhibit B contains HUD's "Important Health Notice" targeting elderly, children and asthma/allergy sufferers who may be at a greater risk. Such a classification covers a minimum of 54 million persons or approximately 19% of the 2000 census for children and elderly, and millions more beyond this for allergy sufferers between the children and elderly classifications. It is recognized that there are allergy sufferers in the children and elderly groupings.

Notwithstanding the need to revise the definition of manufactured homes, when and if the indoor air standard of 0.1 ppm is established, it should be applicable to conventional as well as manufactured homes per the findings of Dr. Randolph and Drs. Ritchie and Lehnen covered in Part 1.

PART V - RECOMMENDATIONS

A. It is time for the reader to stop Corporate America from controlling your destiny and that of your family by sitting down and writing a letter or post card to your Representative in Congress citing "Wake Up, America" and demanding an indoor air standard of 0.1 parts per million (ppm) maximum concentration of hazardous indoor chemicals in conventional, manufactured and trailer homes. Only a flood of letters or post cards can stop Corporate America with its campaign contributions resulting in weak regulations or none at all where they are needed. Address your envelope or post card as follows:

Rep. (name)
House Office Building (Rayburn, Longworth or Cannon)
Washington, D.C. 20515

While this standard, if enacted, would automatically ban particleboard in all types of home construction, the reader could ask for this ban to ensure that this material would no longer kill innocent people.

B. While it would take years for Congress to act on behalf of consumers, and given the unhealthy homes being offered in the marketplace, the reader should avoid particleboard in new home construction or remodeling, preferring instead plywood, wafer board or oriented strand board (OSB) containing less formaldehyde. In addition, avoid wall-to-wall carpeting with exception of "Berber", "Shaw", "Mohawk", and "Alladin" products that should contain a safe "facsimile latex" for use in manufacturing. If the reader suspects the wrong purchase of any products in the past six years, he or she should ventilate indoor areas whenever weather permits, to avoid the cumulative effects of chemical offgassing.

C. While manufactured home dealerships will continue to avoid posting of the HUD-required Health Notice, request your congressman to propose a bill requiring an annual report by HUD stating how many dealerships have been inspected and how many Notices were found missing.

D. With reference to Part II, Federal workers in the 50 states and District of Columbia who are aware of exposure to recycled particleboard furniture, should write to his or her congressman or Delegate for D.C. requesting action to revise Executive Order 13101 issued in 1998 to exclude particleboard from recycling efforts, and to replace all recycled furniture with furniture not containing particleboard.

E. Last but not least, politicians of both major political parties guilty of contributing to lax regulations resulting in the deaths of thousands of innocent Americans while pleasing Corporate America for financial gain, and occupying key positions in the legislative and executive branches of government, are hereby notified that the readers of this publication will not stand for inaction and excuses for not enacting appropriate laws and regulations to establish an indoor air standard of 0.1 ppm maximum concentration of hazardous indoor chemicals in all types of homes; and the banning of particleboard in the construction of all types of homes as well as its use for all types of furniture. Inaction and excuses will hopefully result in defeat of those politicians when running for re-election.

EXHIBIT A

EXCERPT: P. 31996, Federal Register of August 9, 1984

Federal Register / Vol. 49.

DEPARTMENT OF HOUSING AND URBAN DEVELOPMENT

Office of the Assistant Secretary for Housing-Federal Housing Commissioner

24 CFR Part 3280

[Docket No. R-84-1068; FR 1637]

Manufactured Home Construction and Safety Standarts

AGENCY: Office of the Assistant Secretary for Housing-Federal Housing Commissioner, HUD.

ACTION: Final rule. (Background)

SUMMARY: HUD is revising its Manufactured Home Construction and Safety Standards to improve the safety and quality of manufactured homes. Standards limiting permissible amounts of formaldehyde emissions from plywood and particleboard are being added. Standards relating to fire safety are being revised.

EFFECTIVE DATE: October 29, 1984.
II. Formaldehyde Regulation

A. General

The Department has concluded that a Federal Standard designed to limit formaldehyde emissions in manufactured homes should be adopted. The formaldehyde rule is a product standard which limits the level of formaldehyde emitted from particleboard floor decking and cabinetry and from interior plywood installed in manufactured homes. The rule requires that formaldehyde emissions not exceed 0.2 parts per million (ppm) from plywood and 0.3 ppm from particleboard as measured by a specific air chamber test. Generally, manufactured home manufacturers must use only particleboard and plywood that comply with these emissions standards and are certified as meeting the standards.

EXCERPT: P 31998, Federal Register of August 9, 1984

B. Targeted Ambient Level

The Department has concluded that an indoor ambient formaldehyde level of 0.4 ppm provides reasonable protection to manufactured home occupants. The Department has determined that the plywood and particleboard standards will result in indoor ambient formaldehyde levels of not greater than 0.4 ppm when: (1) The indoor temperature does not exceed 77° F: (2) the indoor relative humidity level does not exceed 50%; (3) the homes ventilation rate is at least 0.5 air change per hour (ACH); and (4) there are no other major emitters of formaldehyde, such as MDF, installed in the home.

1. Home Conditions

There was a considerable amount of disagreement in the comments concerning how often the O.4 ppm level would be exceeded in the home. Many commenters stated that, given the conditions which exist to achieve a 0.4 ppm ambient level, it is likely that homes constructed with plywood and particleboard that meet the standard will, at times, exceed 0.4 ppm. Some of these commenters said that the 0.4 ppm target would be exceeded quite often, especially in the summer months. One source expressed the opinion that, even if the stated environmental conditions are met, the ambient level in the home will be 0.5 ppm. Still other commenters said that the proposed product standards leave an adequate margin to achieve 0.4 ppm in the home, even if there are other sources of formaldehyde present or if the air exchange rate is less than 0.5 ACH.

(a) *Temperature and humidity conditions.* There was general agreement in the comments that increases in temperature and humidity increase formaldehyde emission rates. This was of particular concern to commenters from the southern States. They stated that 77° F and 50% relative humidity are exceeded often in their States. A major consumer organizations reported that these temperature and humidity conditions would be exceeded most often in States with the highest manufactured home populations, citing Florida, Texas, and California specifically. One State claimed that the Department was ignoring its statutory mandate by not considering the geographical location of the regulated homes in developing the formaldehyde rule. [See 42 U.S.C. 5403(f)(3).]

EXCERPT: P. 31999, Federal Register of August 9, 1984

2. Health Effects

There was considerable disagreement in the comments regarding the adequacy of 0.4 ppm to protect manufactured home occupants from discomfort and from acute and chronic health effects. Some commenters stated generally that this level is too high to protect home occupants' health. Others said that there is ample medical and scientific evidence to support the 0.4 ppm level. Several commented that the target 0.4 ppm level is obsolete, pointing out that the Department's product standards do not reduce levels below those voluntarily achieved by the industry.

HUD believes that the product standards will result in a 0.4 ppm indoor level under the specific conditions and that this level, given economic considerations, is reasonable. The Department realizes that this targeted level will not be achieved at all times. However, the currently available medical and scientific evidence does not adequately establish the effect on health benefits of a level below 0.4 ppm. In any event, it is not possible to implement a formaldehyde standard that will protect the entire population.

(a) Acute health effects and threshold levels. The extent, intensity, and duration of symptoms

caused by exposure to formaldehyde vary, depending on the individual and the level of formaldehyde in the home. Common complaints include eye, nose, and throat irritation, persistent cough, skin irritation, nausea, headache, dizziness, and respiratory distress. The symptoms usually diminish or disappear when the individual leaves the home.

Several commenters stated that the 0.4 ppm target ambient level is too high to protect the majority of manufactured home occupants from odor and irritation. Consumers wrote letters relating their personal experiences with formaldehyde, in some cases attaching letters from physicians and results of tests measuring the levels of formaldehyde in their homes. These letters chronicled the occurrence of acute symptoms at levels as low as 0.15 ppm. A comment from one State agency reported that the agency received many complaints from people in homes where formaldehyde levels were measured between 0.1 ppm and 0.4 ppm. Another State agency submitted the results of a study it funded that preliminarily analyzed acute symptomatology and found no association with formaldehyde concentration in indoor air.

Other commenters submitted evidence showing varying degrees of functional disturbance and response to low levels of formaldehyde. Several commenters stated that 20% of the population will experience slight irritation at levels from 0.05 ppm to 0.5ppm. A major industry trade association said that the irritation threshold is between 0.8 ppm to 1.2 ppm and that the general population will not experience adverse effects from exposure to 0.5 ppm formaldehyde.

The Department has concluded that there is insufficient medical and scientific evidence to substantiate more than minimal health benefits when formaldehyde levels are reduced below 0.4 ppm.

EXCERPT: P. 32000, Federal Register of August 9, 1984

(c) *Chronic health effects and carcinogenicity.* Respiratory illnesses reported to be caused by chronic formaldehyde exposure include difficulty in breathing and other asthma-like symptoms, persistent cough, and chest congestion. Further, statistically significant incidences of nasal cancer (squamous cell carcinoma) occurred in rats exposed to 15.0 ppm formaldehyde gas (Final Report: A Chronic Inhalation of Toxicology Study on Rats and Mice Exposed to Formaldehyde. CIIT/Batelle Laboratories, 1981).

In terms of chronic health effect, the comments primarily focused on the carcinogenic risk posed by exposure to formaldehyde. Generally, the Commenters were divided into those who believe that formaldehyde should be presumed to be a human carcinogen and those who maintain that there are sufficient human epidemiological and animal studies to conclude that formaldehyde presents a cancer risk to humans. A State Attorney General criticized the Department for failing to take a position on this issue, citing a report from the Congressional Office of Technology Assessment which concluded that, in the absence of epidemiological data concerning a substance's effect on humans, bioessays on carcinogenicity in animals should be used to identify potential human carcinogens.

Among those commenters who presumed that formaldehyde is a human carcinogen, there was disagreement regarding the extent of the risk presented by exposure to a level of 0.4 ppm. Some commenters said that using the highest level of exposure in the CIIT study, 15.0 ppm, and applying a safety factor of 100, there is a significant level of risk at 0.15 ppm. These commenters asserted that this method of calculation is conservative because, when no threshold is known, a 1000-fold or greater safety factor often is used. This conclusion was used as a basis for recommending that the appropriate ambient formaldehyde level is no more than 0.1 ppm. Other commenters said that the animal and human studies performed to date establish that the cancer risk at 0.4 ppm formaldehyde is virtually nonexistent. A large compilation of studies and reports was submitted by the Formaldehyde institute showing that there is no basis, as this time, for treating formaldehyde as a human carcinogen.

On May 23, 1984, the Environmental Protection Agency designated formaldehyde for expedited regulatory Substances Control act (TSCA) (49FR 21870). In the publication, EPA action under section 4(f) of the TSCA stated that there may be a reasonable basis to conclude that formaldehyde presents a significant risk of widespread harm to humans from cancer. The EPA determined that there are animal data on formaldehyde that can be used to assess the human cancer risk. One of the exposure categories to which the section 4(f) decision applies is the exposure associated with residence in manufactured homes.

In addition, The Executive Office of the President, Office of Science and Technology Policy, issued a draft document containing guidelines to be used by regulatory agencies in assessing cancer risks from chemicals (40 FR 21594) (May 22, 1984). The Department has reviewed these guidelines and will evaluate them further when the final report is issued.

The Department will monitor the EPA's regulatory progress closely. In its May 23rd publication, the EPA clearly stated that its decision does not mean that the agency believes that formaldehyde presents short-term emergency risks. Further, the EPA stated that "information available to the Agency does not indicate that people should substantially change their habits if they are being exposed to some level of formaldehyde." Therefore, the Department does not believe it would be appropriate to change the formaldehyde standards when the EPA reaches a final regulatory decision and may change the standards if the basis for EPA's findings show that these standards are not adequate to protect the health of manufactured home occupants.

Because the scientific community has not resolved the human carcinogenic issue, HUD has not taken a position as to whether formaldehyde causes cancer in humans. (See the discussion of this issue in the proposed rule (48 FR 37178.)

EXCERPT: Pp. 32002-32003, Federal Register of August 9, 1984

H. Cost Assessment

The Act requires that the Secretary consider the probable effect of any standard on the cost of the manufactured home to the public (42U. S.C.5003(f)(4)). Several sources commented on this obligation. Some generally criticized the Department's efforts to assess the cost of all the proposed revisions. Others focused on the cost associated with the formaldehyde standards. One commenter stated that the Department's cost analysis had two major deficiencies: Health impacts which could not be quantified were given little, if any, weight, and a number of potentially viable control technologies were not considered. Another stated that the HUD proposed standards would do little to reduce formaldehyde levels below those voluntarily achieved by the industry and that it is HUD's obligation to promulgate regulations which will further reduce formaldehyde levels to the extent feasible within economic constrains. A similar comment said that the cost of the proposed standard is essentially zero and that, therefore, a considerable amount could be spent without pricing manufactured homes out of their current market. Another commenter said that it is not possible to develop an appropriate formaldehyde standard because the costs are not known and the benefits are not ascertainable.

Some commenters addressed the targeted 0.4 ppm level, several saying that there was no apparent economic or technical justification for choosing this level. The manufactured home industry disagreed and provided specific cost information which showed that the cost of the proposed standard would be $27.04 for the average single-section home and $36.48 for the average multi-section home. These figures were based on a cost study funded by the Formaldehyde Institute which calculated that the annual costs of testing as proposed would result in cost increases of $26.00 per 1000 square feet of plywood and $5.20 per 1000 square feet of particleboard. According to the Formaldehyde Institute's contractor, this would raise the cost of the average manufactured home $288.

Finally, other commenters concentrated on the costs of lowering the formaldehyde standard to achieve less than 0.4 ppm in the home. Several commenters generally stated that the Department had not demonstrated that further reducing or eliminating formaldehyde in the home would be significantly more expensive. One source said that plywood wall paneling which emits 0.15 ppm formaldehyde currently is available at no additional cost.

EXHIBIT B

24 CFR Ch. XX (4-1-95 Edition)

§3280.309 Health Notice on formaldehyde emissions.

(a) Each manufactured home shall have a Health Notice on formaldehyde emissions prominently displayed in a temporary manner in the kitchen (i.e., countertop or exposed cabinet face). The Notice shall read as follows:

IMPORTANT HEALTH NOTICE

Some of the building materials used in this home emit formaldehyde. Eye, nose, and throat irritation, headache, nausea, and a variety of asthma-like symptoms, including shortness of breath, have been reported as a result of formaldehyde exposure. Elderly persons and young children, as well as anyone with a history of asthma, allergies, or lung problems, may be at greater risk. Research is continuing on the possible long-term effects of exposure to formaldehyde.

Reduced ventilation resulting from energy efficiency standards may allow formaldehyde and other contaminants to accumulate in the indoor air. Additional ventilation to dilute the indoor air may be obtained from a passive or mechanical ventilation system offered by the manufacturer. Consult your dealer for information about the ventilation options offered with this home.

High indoor temperatures and humidity raise formaldehyde levels. When a home is to be located in areas subject to extreme summer temperatures, an air-conditioning system can be used to control indoor temperature levels. Check the comfort cooling certificate to determine if this home had been equipped or designed for the installation of an air-conditioning system.

If you have any questions regarding the health effects of formaldehyde, consult your doctor or local health department.

(b) The Notice shall be legible and typed using letters at least ¼ inch in size. The title shall be typed using letters at least ¾ inch in size.

(c) The Notice shall not be removed by any party until the entire sales transaction has been completed (refer to part 3282 – Manufactured

Home Procedural and Enforcement Regulations for provisions regarding a sales transaction).

(d) A copy of the Notice shall be included in the Consumer Manual (refer to part 3283 – Manufactured Home Consumer Manual Requirements).

[49 FR 32012, Aug. 9, 1984, as amended at 54 FR 46049, Nov. 1, 1989; 58 FR 55007, Oct. 25, 1993]

Source: Title 24, Code of Federal Regulations

EXHIBIT C

OCCUPANT SYMPTOM/HEALTH PROBLEM CHECKLIST

For each resident indicate with a check persistent or recurring symptoms/health problems which cannot be associated with any readily diagnosed illness such as cold, flu, etc.

Symptoms   **Occupant's Name**

Eye irritation
Eye infection
Dry/sore throat
Cough
Excessive phlegm production
Runny nose
Sinus congestion
Sinus infection
Bronchial pneumonia

Shortness of breath
Wheezing
Asthmatic attacks
Bronchitis
Headaches
Disturbed concentration
Dizziness
Unusual fatigue
Depression
Difficulty in sleeping
Rashes
Nosebleed
Nasal Sores
Nausea
Diarrhea/loose stool
Chest pain
Abdominal pain
Menstrual problems
Unusual thirst

SOURCE:
Indoor Air Quality Notes:
Formaldehyde – Our Homes and Health
Summer, 1989
By: Thad Godish, Ph.D, Director
Indoor Air Quality Research Laboratory
Dept. of Natural Resources
Ball State University
Muncie, Indiana 47306

About The Author

He was born on Capitol Hill in Washington, D.C. in 1926. After high school, he volunteered for the U.S. Navy in 1944 and was assigned to a Navy Reefer for supply runs from Pearl Harbor to Okinawa during the ongoing battle there. On one of the return trips, he was in a typhoon in the China Sea, and aboard the only ship in the convoy to survive.

Later, he was shipwrecked and assigned to the aircraft carrier U.S.S. Hancock. On departing, his commendation stated "The loss of this man's services to the U.S. Navy is to be regretted."

After the war, he worked for Public Accountants and attended night school. In 1947, he married a former Lady Marine who lived next door on

Capitol Hill. In 1950, he was awarded a Bachelor of Science degree from Columbus University of Washington, D.C., and later attended Georgetown University's School of Foreign Service.

He entered Federal service in 1956 at the National Security Agency, and later, the Department of Defense. In 1962, he transferred to the Federal Aviation Administration and was awarded a Presidential Citation in 1965 for saving millions of dollars in aircraft maintenance. In 1972, he was awarded the designation Certified Internal Auditor. He retired in 1985 and devoted most of his time to research.